The 10 Day Detox with REAL Food

by

Anne Angelone

TABLE OF CONTENT

ISBN-13:
978-1484091050

ISBN-10:
1484091051

Disclaimer

This program manual is not intended to provide medical advice or to take the place of medical advice and treatment from your personal physician

Readers are advised to consult their own doctors or other qualified health professionals regarding the treatment of medical conditions

The author, shall not be held liable or responsible for any misunderstanding or misuse of the information contained in this program manual or for any loss, damage, or injury caused or alleged to be caused directly or indirectly by any treatment, action, or application of any food or food source discussed in this program manual

The statements in this program manual have not been evaluated by the U.S Food and Drug Administration

This information is not intended to diagnose, treat, cure, or prevent any disease.

To request permission for reproduction or inquire about consulting about autoimmunity, please contact:

Anne Angelone, Licensed Acupuncturist

website: www.anneangelone.com

INTRODUCTION

This 10 Day Detox program is based on the exciting field of nutritional science called Nutrigenomics which studies how food/nutrients regulate inflammatory gene expression and thus suppress the inflammatory response. The process of silencing inflammatory gene suppression via certain nutrients is called DNA methylation. Nutrigenomics makes the case for positioning potent nutrients over the epigenome (the area just above the genes) to promote optimal gene expression. The idea is to pack in the nutrients required to increase the odds of dimming down inflammatory genes that may have already been turned on. Research has shown that our genes are very much affected by the epigenome. In order to nurture the best possible genetic expression, you must start shoring up your epigenome with the best possible nutrients!

What foods create the best possible cell signaling and genetic expression?

REAL Food: mostly greens, beneficial fats, the least allergenic grains, grass fed animal and fish protein. Shoring up the body with nutrients for detoxification and DNA protection is the key to health and what this program is aiming to do. "Ultra Clear Plus" is suggested in this guide as a recommendation but not required. Ultra Clear Plus contains nutrients for liver detoxification and provides a full complement of protein, fat and carbs plus extra nutrients. It's refreshing and can be mixed with water or nut milk for a snack or meal replacement. The goal of the 10 Day Detox is to eliminate inflammatory foods and facilitate better gene expression.

Excellent nutrition and absorption are really the cornerstones of maintaining great health. The digestive system is an integral part of the immune system and plays a significant role in a persons sense of well being. Leaky gut is very common today and can cause bloating, heartburn, gas, constipation, diarrhea, or pain. However, many people with leaky gut have no digestive symptoms at all.

One of the most common causes of leaky gut is eating gluten, the protein found in wheat, rye, barley, spelt, and other wheat-like grains. Wheat today is not like the wheat from past generations. It has been genetically altered, processed, and stored in ways that make it very damaging to people's guts. Sometimes simply removing gluten from the diet can profoundly relieve allergy symptoms by allowing the gut to recover and repair. Because leaky gut leads to food intolerances and food allergies, you are encouraged to eliminate other foods, such as dairy, eggs, or other grains.

Another factor that contributes to leaky gut and allergy symptoms is an imbalance of gut bacteria. The digestive tract holds several pounds of bacteria that play a large role in immune function. When the bad bacteria overwhelm the good, inflammation and allergies result. Leaky gut repair includes nurturing your beneficial bacteria with probiotics and fermented foods to improve digestion.

Chronic stress also weakens and inflames the digestive tract, causing leaky gut. Stress doesn't just have to come from a stressful lifestyle or lack of sleep, although those certainly play a role. Eating a diet high in sugar and processed foods is stressful to the body, as is an unmanaged autoimmune disease, or hormones that are out of whack and causing miserable PMS or menopausal symptoms.

The 10 Day Detox is a great way to find out what foods may be inflaming you by eliminating all of the major food allergens, including gluten, dairy, corn, soy and nightshade vegetables. Just taking this burden off your digestive tract and immune system will quickly rid your body of inflammation, stiffness and allergic responses while your energy simultaneously skyrockets, your skin clears and your are ready to tackle the world again. Dust off your cells! Learn how you can easily shop for, cook, and eat delicious meals that give your body what it needs to set the foundation for long term health. Detoxification from the major food allergens is step 1. Making small daily changes toward a less inflamed body (essentially more veggies, breathing and mindfulness) will bring the benefit of more sustainable health.

Start today by applying this plan and you will quickly begin receiving the benefits of better digestion and elimination, fewer symptoms of chronic illness, improved concentration, mental focus and clarity, improved mood, increased energy, less congestion, fewer allergic symptoms, less joint pain, increased sense of relaxation and enhanced sleep.

10 Day Detox Guidelines

1. Avoidance of the major food allergens to heal your gut.
2. Eliminate: gluten, corn, soy, dairy, eggs, nightshades.
3. Use extra fiber, digestive enzymes and hydrochloric acid as needed.
4. Drink green smoothies daily.
5. Add beneficial foods
6. Reduce Inflammation with shakes/smoothies
7. Relax: bathe with epsom salt & baking soda; sauna therapy
8. Reintroduce each eliminated food slowly
9. Drink 8 glasses of filtered water each day
10. Liver detox – 1 tablespoon olive oil & 1 tablespoon lemon
11. Raw apple cider vinegar - 1 tablespoon diluted with 1 tablespoon water helps your stomach produce hydrochloric Acid.
12. Easy exercise - 30 minute walk / day
13. Include grass fed organic protein, vegetables and fats 3 meals per day.
14. Drink 8 glasses of water per day and include daily veggie broth.
15. Exercise every day even if it's just swinging your arms for 5 minutes!
16. Relax with an awareness of your breath for 5 minutes per day.

	Foods To Include	Foods To Eliminate
FRUITS	In Season, Organic, Fresh, Apples, apricots, Asian pears, bananas, blueberries, blackberry, boysenberry, cherries, cranberry, figs, grapefruit, kiwi, lemons, limes, melons, nectarine, oranges, peaches, pears, persimmons, plums, pluots, plantains, pomegranate, raspberry, strawberry.	Avoid: Dried and canned fruits, high glycemic fruits: watermelon, mango, pineapple, raisins, grapes, and store bought fruit juice.
VEGETABLES	All fresh raw, steamed, sautéed, juiced, or roasted vegetables. Asparagus, avocado, basil, beet, broccoli, cabbage, carrots, cauliflower, celery, chard, collards, cucumber, green beans, green onion, kale, kohlrabi, kumquats, lettuce, mushroom, mustard, okra, onions, spinach, summer squash, turnips, artichoke hearts, Brussels sprouts, carrots, daikon, zucchini, fennel root, dandelion greens, bell pepper, cabbage.	Corn, tomato, tomato sauce, and any creamed vegetables, salsa; avoid nightshades: Potatoes (not sweet potatoes), all tomatoes, green peppers, chili peppers, eggplants, tomatillos, sweet bell peppers, jalapenos, cayenne, habanero, Anaheim and Serrano, chili peppers in dried powders such as paprika, chili powder, curry powder, cayenne, hot sauces, salsas, goji berries, ashwaganda, tobacco.

LEGUME

All legumes including peas and lentils (except soybeans). Soak overnight to reduce gas.

Avoid:
Soybeans, tofu, tempeh, soy milk, soy sauce, or any products containing soy proteins such as soy cheese and Bragg's Aminos.

BREAD AND GRAINS

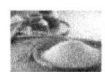

Avoid:
Products made from rice, buckwheat, millet, quinoa, amaranth

Corn, plus all gluten-containing grains and products including wheat, spelt, kamut, barley, rye, oat.

NUTS AND SEEDS

Nuts except peanuts. Almonds, cashews, walnuts, pumpkin seeds, brazil nuts, sunflower seeds, etc., – whole or as a nut butter (preferably organic and/or raw); sprouting or soaking overnight is highly encouraged.

Avoid:
Peanuts, peanut butter.

MEAT

Beef, chicken; quail, squab, duck, goose, turkey, Cornish game hen; pasture-raised lamb, pork, buffalo/bison, goat, emu, ostrich, sausage (without fillers or nightshade spices); liver, kidney, heart, organic sliced meats (gluten, sugar free), uncured nitrate/nitrite-free deli meats and bacon from grass-fed/pastured beef/pork.

Avoid: Processed and canned meats: bacon, fatty cuts of lamb, beef, pork, deli meats, smoked/dried/salted meat and fish. Sausages and deli meats with seed-based or nightshade spices.

WILD FISH

Salmon, mackerel, herring, halibut, shellfish, oysters, cod, tuna, flounder, sardines, hake, skate, trout, red snapper, etc.

Avoid: Whale, shark, swordfish.

Farmed tilapia and catfish quantities should be moderate.

FATS

Extra virgin olive oil, coconut oil, avocado oil, coconut oil, red palm oil, flaxseed, sesame, walnut, hazelnut oil.

Avoid: Margarine, butter, shortening, peanut oil, mayonnaise, any processed hydrogenated oils.

DRINKS

Filtered or distilled water, herbal tea, coffee, mineral water, broths, freshly made veggie juice, green smoothies, kefir water, coconut kefir, kombucha.

Avoid:
Sodas and soft drinks, fruit juice, caffeinated beverages.

SPICES

Ginger, rosemary, basil, cilantro, dill, ginger, lemongrass, peppermint, oregano, parsley, sage, sea, salt, thyme, tarragon, turmeric, spearmint, marjoram, mace, chives, chamomile, chervil, cinnamon, bay leaves, cloves, dill, horseradish, saffron, sea salt.

CONDIMENTS

Apple cider vinegar, Balsamic vinegar, coconut vinegar, Red Boat fish sauce and coconut aminos, wasabi, mustard, horseradish, pesto.

Avoid: Ketchup, relish, soy sauce, BBQ sauce, chutneys, baker's yeast, brewer's yeast.

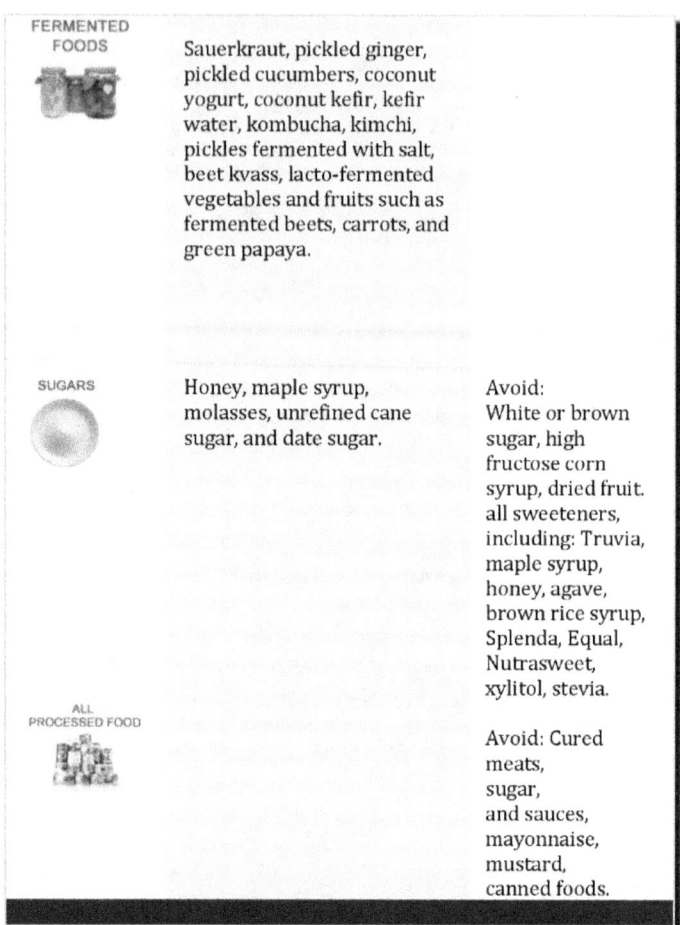

FERMENTED FOODS	Sauerkraut, pickled ginger, pickled cucumbers, coconut yogurt, coconut kefir, kefir water, kombucha, kimchi, pickles fermented with salt, beet kvass, lacto-fermented vegetables and fruits such as fermented beets, carrots, and green papaya.	
SUGARS	Honey, maple syrup, molasses, unrefined cane sugar, and date sugar.	Avoid: White or brown sugar, high fructose corn syrup, dried fruit. all sweeteners, including: Truvia, maple syrup, honey, agave, brown rice syrup, Splenda, Equal, Nutrasweet, xylitol, stevia.
ALL PROCESSED FOOD		Avoid: Cured meats, sugar, and sauces, mayonnaise, mustard, canned foods.

Avoid any food triggers, even if they are fruits and vegetables on the "include list".

THE 10 DAYS

DAY 1

Eliminate all: refined sugars & carbohydrates – anything with added sucrose, high fructose corn syrup, or alcohol (cakes, cookies, candies, pastries, beer, wine, liquor, ice-cream). Caffeinated drinks (sodas, coffee, caffeinated teas with exception of green tea). Artificial colorings, flavorings, sweeteners (packaged, preserved, processed foods).

Start: Ultra Clear Plus– 1 scoop twice today (once in morning, once after a meal).

DAY 2

In addition to eliminating foods listed for Day 1,

Eliminate all: dairy products and eggs.

Continue: Ultra Clear Plus– 1 scoop twice / day.

DAY 3

In addition to eliminating foods listed for Days 1 & 2,

Eliminate all: gluten grains–wheat, oat, rye, barley, spelt, kamut, bulgar as well as corn & corn-derived foods.

Continue: Ultra Clear Plus– 1 scoop twice / day.

Note: Continue to eat quinoa, rice (preferably brown), millet, amaranth and buckwheat.

DAY 4

In addition to eliminating foods listed for Days 1 & 2,

Eliminate all: soy products, and all night shade vegetables including tomatoes, potatoes, eggplant.

Continue: Ultra Clear Plus– 2 scoops twice / day.

DAY 5-10

You're doing great!   Continue: Ultra Clear Plus– 2 scoops twice / day.

DAY 10

Congratulations! You have successfully completed the 10 Day Detox Program!

***For maximum benefit from this program, it is important to **slowly reintroduce the foods**.*

When you start reintroducing foods, if you suspect that you have food allergies try only one new food at a time, and wait **72 hours** to see if you note a reaction. If unsure about a reaction, wait until symptoms recede, and eat only foods that do not cause a reaction. Then ingest the suspicious food again and take note.

The Recipes

PROTEIN SHAKE

Nutritious, cleansing, and anti-inflammatory

- Blend with 1 cup of rice milk/ almond milk / hemp milk / hazelnut milk or water 2 scoops of Ultra-Clear Plus protein powder.
- Optional: Add fruit,1/2 cup, apple, persimmon, pear, kiwi.
- 2 scoops/2x day - 1 in the morning before breakfast and one between meal (breakfast and lunch or lunch and dinner).

ALMOND MILK

Raw almonds (soak overnight)

1. Strain & thoroughly rinse 1 cup of nuts.
2. Put in blender, add 5 cups filtered water & blend.
3. Strain through a thin mesh colander or nut milk bag/cheese cloth.
4. Flavor options add: cinnamon, vanilla, cardamon.
5. Raw cocoa powder; carob.

BREAKFAST

ANNE'S BREAKFAST MUESLI:

- 1 scoop freshly grounded flax
- 1 scoop sesame
- 1 scoop sunflower
- 1 scoop pumpkin
- 1 scoop sliced almonds
- Cut up apples, pears, persimmons

Optional:

Consider adding nut milk / coconut milk, or adding cooked red Bhutanese, millet, red quinoa.

MILLET, ADZUKI BEAN, SWEET POTATO PORRIDGE

- 1 cup millet soaked overnight in 3 cups water
- 1 cup adzuki beans soaked overnight in 3 cups water (sprout them is even better!)
- 1 small sweet potato cubed
- 1/2 teaspoon cinnamon
- 1 tablespoon dried goji berries or raisins (optional)
- 1 teaspoon dulse seaweed (optional)
- 1 tablespoon olive oil
- 3 cups water
- Handful nut or seeds (almonds, cashews, pumpkin seeds, etc.)

If you have a rice cooker or slow cooker then put all the ingredients in and cook. If not, bring all ingredients to a boil in a saucepan, and then turn down to simmer. Cook on low heat for 50 min to 1 hr or until all the liquid is absorbed and it has a porridge-like consistency. Add 1 teaspoon flax seed oil to serve. You can also add 1 tablespoon maple syrup or honey if you want it to be sweeter.

TIP: for maximum absorption of nutrients - sprout your seeds & beans, and soak your grains.

CREAM OF "WHEAT"

- 1/2 cup brown rice
- 1/2 cup buckwheat
- 15 almonds
- 1 tablespoon unsweetened, dried coconut
- Grind until mealy in a coffee grinder.
- Add 1/2 cup amaranth

- Boil 3 cups water and add one cup of the above mixture. Turn heat down to simmer and add:
- 1/2 teaspoon each cinnamon, nutmeg, cloves
- 1 tablespoon goji berries
- 1/4 cup diced apple (ok to leave skin on)
- Cook for 15-20 minutes stirring occasionally to take the lumps out. Should have the consistency of cream of wheat when it is finished. Add to taste:
- 1-2 tablespoon maple syrup
- 2 teaspoon flax seed oil
- 1 tablespoon sunflower seeds

ALMOND FLOUR PANCAKES

- 1 cup almond flour
- 2 eggs
- ¼ cup water
- 1 teaspoon vanilla extract
- 1 tablespoon coconut oil for cooking
- pinch of cinnamon and salt

Whisk the eggs and vanilla in a bowl. add almond flour, cinnamon and a pinch of salt and mix well.

Heat 1 tablespoon of coconut oil, and pour the batter in to make your pancakes at whatever size you like

COCONUT YOGURT

1. Heat 1 quart of unsweetened coconut milk to105F - 110F which will bring the milk temperature closer to the fermenting temperature of 115F to 120F.
2. Add ¼ teaspoon of yogurt starter (GI Pro-health makes a good non-dairy starter) for every 1 quart of milk and give it about 5 long pulses with the blender. Making sure the yogurt starter mixes well with the milk. If you are making two quarts at a time just pour the milk in a bowl and mix starter in with a whisk. You can add more

then 1/4 teaspoon per quart if a very firm yogurt is desired.
3. Plug in your yogurt maker and pour the mixture into your yogurt maker container or containers and ferment for 12 hours.
4. Place in refrigerator for 4 hours then your yogurt is ready to eat.

GREEN SMOOTHIES

- 1/2 a bunch dino kale or swiss chard, cut out stalks
- 1/2 inch ginger
- ½ cup blueberries
- 5 cups of water
- Blend for 5 minutes

Savory Dishes

TIP: Stock up on supplies and prep your veggies & grains (clean, cut, cook).

WINTER VEGETABLES

ROASTED ROOT VEGETABLES

Any root vegetables can be used in this recipe. Root vegetables are high in minerals as well as vitamins.

- 1 turnip (½ cup chopped)
- 1 parsnip (½ cup chopped)
- 1 red onion (½ cup chopped)
- 1/2 celery root (½ cup chopped)
- 1 beet (½ cup chopped)
- 2-3 sweet potatoes (¾ cup chopped)
- 1 sprig fresh rosemary (leaves separated from stalk and chopped coarsely)
- 1 sprig fresh thyme (leaves separated from stalk)
- 2 tablespoon coconut oil and 2 table olive oil
- ½ teaspoon salt

Preheat the oven to 350 degrees F. Put half of the olive oil on the bottom of the medium to large size baking dish. Cut all of the vegetables into roughly the same size pieces and put in the baking dish. Pour the remaining olive oil and sprinkle the garlic, rosemary and thyme over the top tossing with your hands to coat evenly. Crumble the coconut oil over the top.

Put the baking dish in the preheated oven and cook, stirring the vegetables occasionally, until they are tender and golden brown, about 45 minutes. Serve warm.

DARK GREEN STIR FRY

- 1 cup dino kale (chopped)
- 1 cup bok choy (chopped)
- 1/2 cup carrots (diced)
- 1/4 teaspoon pepper
- 1/4 cup vegetable broth ("no-chicken broth")
- 1 tablespoon coconut aminos
- 1 tablespoon olive oil
- 1 wedge lemon
- Salt to taste

WINTER SQUASH WITH SAGE

- 1-2 Winter Squash(any kind!)
- 2 tablespoon olive oil
- Fresh sage
- Fresh thyme
- Pinch salt and pepper
- 1 tablespoon coconut aminos

Preheat oven to 375 degrees F. Cut squash into manageable pieces. Scoop out seeds and rinse so they are clean. Pour 1 tablespoon olive oil in oven pan or other deep dish pan. Put squash in pan and add sage, thyme, salt, pepper, coconut amino's and other 1 tablespoon olive oil. Toss contents. Put into oven for 40-45 minutes taking out to stir at least once. Squash should be soft and easy to pierce with a fork when it's done. Serve with grains and greens!

FABULOUS KALE CHIPS

Servings : 4.

- 1 large bunch of dino kale, stems removed and leaves chopped
- extra virgin olive oil
- sea salt to taste

- garlic powder

Massage Kale with other ingredient and bake at 350 for 15 min. Let cool.

GRILL PAN CHICKEN COLLARD WRAP

Servings : 2.

- 6 collard leaves, cut lengthwise into two large pieces (stems removed)
- carrot, cucumber, celery, cut into sticks
- handful of cilantro, whole or chopped
- avocado, sliced into wedges
- 2 organic chicken breasts coated with olive oil thyme and sea salt

Grill chicken, cut into slices and make a wrap with crunchy veggies inside the collard greens.

TRI-TIP STEAK AND ASPARAGUS

Servings : 3.

- Tri-tip steak (1 pound)
- 1 head of asparagus
- olive oil
- sea salt and pepper
- 2 sprigs of fresh rosemary

Coat everything with olive oil, chopped rosemary, salt and pepper. Grill to perfection.

COCONUT CHICKEN PAILLARD

Servings: 5.

- 5 chicken breasts
- salt and pepper, to taste
- 1/2 cup coconut flour
- 3 TB olive or coconut oil

- 1 cup chicken broth
- 3 TB capers, drained and rinsed
- 4 sprigs fresh thyme

Coat chicken with olive oil, salt and pepper. Then dip in coconut flour. Transfer chicken in a single layer to hot skillet and cook chicken cutlets 3 or 4 minutes on each side with capers and thyme. Add broth and cook for 15 minutes. Serve.

BRAISED GREENS

Servings : 4.

- 2 TB coconut or olive oil
- 2 heads of greens
- 1/2 yellow onion, chopped
- 3 garlic cloves, chopped
- 1 1/2 cup vegetable, chicken, or beef stock
- salt to taste
- 2 TB apple cider vinegar

Sautee onion and garlic until golden brown then add greens, salt and vinegar. Cover with lid slightly ajar and let the greens cook down for 30 minutes.

SWEET POTATO FRIES

Servings : 4.

- 3 medium sweet potatoes, washed and peeled
- 3 TB coconut oil
- 1 1/2 tsp cumin
- 1 TB salt or to taste

Coat sweet potatoes with oil cumin, salt. Spread on a baking sheet and bake at 425 for 20 minutes.

CARMELIZED BRUSSELS SPROUTS

Servings : 4.

- 1 lb Brussels sprouts
- 3 TBS balsamic vinegar
- 3 TBS olive oil
- black pepper

Sautee sprouts in olive oil on low heat until tender. Increase to high heat and add balsamic vinegar, stir for 30 seconds, turn off flame and season with salt and pepper to taste

GRILLED BALSAMIC PORK TENDERLOIN

Servings : 6.

- 8 garlic cloves, coarsely chopped
- 1 tablespoon fresh oregano, finely chopped
- 1 tablespoon fresh thyme, finely chopped
- 1 tablespoon fresh rosemary, finely chopped
- 1 teaspoon salt
- 1/2 teaspoon pepper
- 1/4 cup balsamic vinegar
- 1/2 cup olive oil
- 2 one pound pork tenderloins
- Marinade pork for up to 24 hours in above ingredients.

Grill to perfection. Serve.

CILANTRO LIME ROAST CHICKEN

Servings : 2-4.

- 1 whole chicken, 6 lbs.
- 1 lime, zested & juiced
- 1/2 bunch cilantro
- 3 green onions, chopped
- 6 cloves garlic, peeled
- 1/4 cup olive oil

- 1 TBSP coconut oil
- salt

Chop and mix ingredients, rub chicken. Bake at 400 for 45 minutes.

BEEF STEW

Servings : Makes large stew.

- grass-fed beef brisket 3 Lbs.
- 10 garlic cloves, peeled
- salt and pepper
- 1 bay leaf
- 1 ½ cups beef broth
- 8 cups of your favorite veggies (leeks, carrots, celery, onions).

Cut slits into beef and add a peeled garlic clove in each. Sprinkle salt and pepper and rub beef. Chop up your veggies and add all ingredients to the slow cooker. Set on high for 4 hours or low for 8 hours.

CROCK POT CHICKEN

Servings : 6.

- 2.5 lbs boneless, skinless chicken thighs
- 3 parsnips
- 3 carrots
- 4 celery stalks
- 1 red onion
- 10-12 whole garlic cloves
- 1/4 cup coconut oil
- 1 cup chicken broth
- 1 TB dried thyme
- 1 TB sage
- sea salt and black pepper to taste

Add everything to your crock pot and let cook on high for 4 hours.

SAUTEED KALE

Servings : 4.

- 2 bunches of kale, leaves pulled off, discard stems
- 1 shallot, finely chopped
- 2 cloves garlic, finely chopped
- 1 TB olive oil

Sautee garlic and shallots in olive oil until golden brown, add in kale until tender.

GINGER SALMON AND BROCCOLI

Servings : 4.

- 1 head broccoli, cut into florets
- 2 TB coconut oil
- salt and pepper to taste
- 1 pound salmon
- squeeze of lemon
- ¼ bunch fresh cilantro
- 1 TBSP ginger, chopped
- 2 TBS coconut aminos

Cover salmon with coconut oil, cilantro, ginger, coconut aminos and a squeeze of lemon.

Grill pan to perfection and serve with steamed broccoli.

NORI CHIPS

Servings : 1.

- 3 nori sheets
- olive oil
- sea salt
- season with onion or garlic powder

Preheat oven to 350. Cut Nori sheets into four and place on baking sheet. Brush or massage nori with oil. Add sea salt and whatever spices you choose. Bake for 15 minutes. Let cool.

Desserts

BERRY ICE CREAM

Servings : 4.

- 1 pint of blueberries or your favorites
- 1/2 cup coconut milk
- 1 tsp vanilla extract

Blend everything in your food processor until smooth and place in freezer.

RASPBERRIES WITH BALSAMIC AND COCONUT MILK

Servings : 2.

- 40 Raspberries
- 2 TB balsamic vinegar
- dash of black pepper
- coconut milk

Cover raspberries in a bowl with 2 TBS of balsamic and let sit for 15 minutes. Grind in pepper, stir and drizzle with coconut milk.

Fish Recipes

GARLIC DILL SALMON

Servings : 2.

- 2 salmon fillets
- 5 cloves garlic, crushed
- olive oil - enough to coat the salmon
- dried dill, and ground black pepper to taste
- the juice from 1 lemon

Mix garlic with dill, olive oil, lemon and coat the salmon. Grill pan to perfection.

BAKED TILAPIA WITH LEMON AND FRESH HERBS

Servings : 4.

- 1 shallot, finely chopped
- 4 tilapia fillets
- 4 teaspoons olive oil
- sea salt and pepper
- 1 teaspoon finely chopped fresh thyme leaves
- ½ TBSP chopped parsley
- ½ TBSP fresh cilantro
- 1 teaspoon salt
- finely grated zest of 2 lemons

Mix herbs and seasonings with olive oil. Add Lemon zest and spread half of seasoning over fish. Place fish in broiler pan lined with parchment paper. Broil in pre-heated broiler 2 inches from heat for 3 minutes. Turn fish, applying remaining seasoning and broil for 3-5 minutes. Serve.

BROILED HALIBUT [OR ANY FRESH/LOCAL/WILD FISH]:

- 2 lb halibut, 1 inch thick
- 1/3 cup olive oil
- 1/2 tablespoon salt
- 1/4 tablespoon pepper
- 1/4 tablespoon thyme
- 1/8 tablespoon tarragon
- 1/4 tablespoon parsley
- tablespoon lemon juice
- 1 cup quinoa

Good baked, broiled on top of any fish. Use two cups water to one cup quinoa. Bring water and quinoa to a boil, stirring occasionally. Cover and simmer for 7-10 minutes.

Mix herbs and seasonings with olive oil. Add Lemon juice slowly. Spread half of seasoning over fish. Place fish in broiler pan lined with parchment paper. Broil in pre-heated broiler 2 inches from heat for 3 minutes. Turn fish, applying remaining seasoning and broil for 3-5 minutes. Serve on platter over quinoa and spoon sauce from the pan over fish.

PUMPKIN SEED PESTO & FISH

- 2 cups unsalted hulled (green) pumpkin seeds
- 6 tablespoon extra-virgin olive oil, divided
- 1/2 tablespoon sea salt
- 1/4 cup water
- 2 tablespoon fresh lemon juice, or to taste
- 4 garlic gloves, smashed
- 1 cup coarsely chopped fresh cilantro
- 1/2 tablespoon parsley, dried
- 1 1/2 lb. fish fillets, whatever is in season, wild, local, sustainable

Preheat oven to 375 F. Toss pumpkin seeds with 2 tablespoons olive oil and sea salt. Roast 10-15 minutes.

Allow to cool. Combine cooled seeds in a food processor with water, lemon juice, garlic, cilantro, and remaining 4 tablespoons oil.

Pulse until mixture forms a coarse paste. Taste and adjust seasoning with salt and pepper. Top fish with pesto mixture and let sit 15-30 minutes. Bake skin side down on oiled grate with grill lit closed about 10 minutes. Use a metal spatula to loosen fish from skin and remove fillets to serving platter.

Salads

RICE SALAD

- 2 cups brown rice, red bhutanese cooked
- 1/3 cup toasted sesame seeds
- 3 tablespoons minced fresh coriander or regular parsley
- 1/2 cup sauerkraut
- 1/4 cup minced celery (use tender, inside stalks)
- 1/4 cup minced green onion
- Olive Oil

Combine ingredients, adding just enough oil to lightly coat vegetables. Additional salt is not needed—the sauerkraut will provide enough.

MIXED GREEN SALAD WITH GINGER SESAME DRESSING

GINGER SESAME DRESSING

- 1/2 cup flaxseed oil
- 1/3 cup raw apple cider vinegar
- 1/4 cup coconut aminos
- 1/2 cup water
- 2 tablespoon sesame oil fresh ginger, grated

MIXED GREENS & SEEDS

- 12 cup (4-5 oz bags) lettuce mix
- 1/2 cup pumpkin seeds
- 1/4 cup sesame seeds
- 2 tablespoon pure hawaiian spirulina

POWER SALAD:

- 1 cup butter lettuce
- 1 cup spinach
- 1/2 cup dino kale (shredded)
- 1/4 cup parsley

- 1/4 cup sprouts (sunflower, broccoli, alfalfa, etc.)
- 1/8 cup fresh basil
- 1/8 cup carrots (diced or shredded)
- 1/8 cup celery (diced)
- 1 avocado (depending on size)
- Small handful pine nuts, sunflower seeds or pumpkin seeds

DRESSING:

- 1/4 cup olive oil
- 1 tablespoon lemon juice (fresh if possible)
- 1 teaspoon balsamic vinegar
- 1teaspoon honey
- Salt and pepper to taste

TIP: Prepare certain foods (veggies, grains, meats) in advance in bulk, so you can whip different dishes easily. Be creative and most of all, have fun!!

BEET SALAD

- 1 lb. beets
- 1 onion, peeled and chopped
- 1 tablespoon lemon juice
- 1 tablespoon chopped parsley
- 1/4 cup olive oil
- 1/4 tablespoon cayenne pepper
- Salt & ground black pepper

Place the beets in a large pot and cover with 3 cups of water, and bring to boil. Remove and let cool, then skin. Dice the beets; add the onions, olive oil, lemon juice, salt, ground peeper, and cayenne pepper, mix well and pour into a serving dish. Sprinkle parsley over it and serve warm or cold.

Soups

CARROT GINGER SOUP

- 4 lbs carrots, peeled and cut into small pieces
- 1 bunch green onions
- 3 tablespoon olive oil
- 2 teaspoon ground cumin
- 5 tablespoons mixed chopped parsley and cilantro
- 1 tablespoon lemon juice
- 1/4 red pepper flakes
- Pinch of cayenne pepper
- Pinch of ginger
- Water
- Pinch salt & ground pepper

In a large pot, mix the oil, onions, carrots, herbs, and all spices. Saute for 5 minutes, cover with water, and bring to boil. Reduce the heat, add lemon juice, red pepper flakes, and let simmer until the carrots are soft. Remove from heat, and puree the whole in a blender until very smooth. If soup too thick, thin with water, taste and adjust seasoning as needed.

CURRIED PARSNIP SOUP

- 1/4 cup olive oil
- 1 large onion, chopped
- 2 cloves garlic, crushed
- 1 teaspoon ground turmeric
- 1/2 teaspoon ground cumin
- 1 1/4 parsnips, peeled and chopped
- 2 apples, peeled, cored and chopped
- 4 cups vegetable/ chicken stock
- Salt and freshly ground black pepper, to taste

Warm oil in large saucepan over medium heat. Add onion and garlic and cook untio onion softens, about 2 minutes. Stir in turmeric, cumin, ginger and chilli pepper, and cook for 3 minutes, stirring occasionally. Add parsnips and apples and stir well. Stir in vegetable stock and season with salt and pepper. Bring mixtures to a boil over high heat, then reduce heat to a simmer. Cover and simmer until parsnips are soft, about 30-40 minutes.

Remove soup from heat and transfer to a large bowl. Work in batches, ladle into a food processor/blender and process until smooth, about 20 seconds. Return soup to the saucepan and heat through over medium heat, about 5 minutes, serves 6.

SQUASH & BEAN SOUP

- 2 tablespoons olive oil
- 3 scallions, finely sliced
- 12 oz carrots, peeled and sliced
- 5 oz rutabaga, peeled and cubed
- 1 lb butternut squash, peeled and cubed
- 6 oz cooked cannelloni beans
- 6 cups of veggie or chicken stock
- 1 bay leaf
- 4 tablespoons chopped fresh mint, for garnish
- 2 tablespoons chopped cilantro leaves, for garnish

Warm olive oil in a large saucepan over medium heat. Add scallions, carrots, rutabaga, squash and chili pepper and cook until veggies soften slightly, about 6 minutes. Add beans, stock, bay leaf and cilantro. Bring to boil. Cover, reduce heat to low and cook until veggies are tender, about 15 minutes.

Working in batches, puree soup in a food processor. Return soup to the pan and heat through, about 3 minutes. Garnish with herbs and serve immediately.

STEAMED ARTICHOKE

Trim the sharp tips of the artichoke leaves off and rinse the artichoke. Place the artichoke in steamer and squeeze the juice of ½ a lemon over the top and sprinkle with herbs or sea salt to taste. Better yet, fill in leaves with a crude pesto of parsley, garlic and kalamata olives. Steam for 45 minutes.

BAKED YAM

Preheat oven to 350 degrees. Scrub and rinse yam "skin". Place into oven and bake for 45 minutes. (The skin is delicious to eat and adds fiber).

BROWN LENTILS

Soak small brown lentils 8-10 hours (overnight). You may use canned beans rather than dried if you prefer. Drain and rinse the beans. Add one part bean to two parts water. Cook for 1 hour. Chop 3 green scallion and 3 stalks of celery and herb or sea salt to taste. Squeeze fresh lemon juice over the beans.

NUTMEG AND CINNAMON BAKED BUTTERNUT SQUASH

Preheat oven to 350 degrees. Cut off the stem and slice down the middle. Scoop out seeds and place the squash and seeds into a baking dish with a small amount of water. Sprinkle with nutmeg and cinnamon. Bake for 45 minutes.

BLACK BEANS

Soak black beans 8-10 hours (overnight). You may use canned beans rather than dried if you prefer. Drain and rinse the beans. Add one part bean to two parts water. Cook for 1 hour. Chop 1 bunch of fresh cilantro and add ¼ teaspoon of cumin or chili powder and herb or sea salt to taste. Squeeze fresh lime juice over the beans.

SESAME WHITE QUINOA

Use one part grain to two parts vegetable stock. Add 1 teaspoon of oregano, 1 teaspoon of thyme, 3 fresh sage leaves and herb or sea salt to taste to the cooking water. Bring to a boil and then simmer for 20 minutes. When the grain is fully cooked, add 1 chopped sweet red pepper, 1 chopped red onion and 1 bunch of freshly chopped basil leaves. Garnish with roasted un-hulled sesame seeds.

SUNFLOWER WILD RICE

Add one part wild rice to two parts vegetable stock and herb or sea salt to taste. Simmer for 30 minutes or until done. Add freshly chopped Arugula greens and 1 teaspoon of toasted sunflower seeds.

COOKED AMARANTH GRAIN

Lightly toast amaranth grain in a pan. Use one part grain to two parts water. Bring to a gentle boil and then simmer for 30 minutes. Add fresh fruit when ready to eat. Add frozen, dried fruit and/or spices a few minutes into the cooking time.

OREGANO-BASIL RED QUINOA

Use one part grain to two parts vegetable stock or water. Add 1 tablespoon of oregano and herb or sea salt to taste to the cooking water and simmer for 20 minutes. When the grain is fully cooked, turn off the heat and add a small amount of olive oil, 3 cloves of chopped garlic, and one bunch of freshly chopped basil leaves. Cover and let stand for 5 minutes.

MILLET SUNFLOWER PATTIES

Use one part grain to two parts vegetable stock or water. Add herb or sea salt to taste to the cooking water. Cook for 30 minutes. While the millet is cooking, puree 3 carrots, 1 bunch of fresh parsley or basil leaves and 2 cloves of garlic. When the millet is fully cooked, turn off the heat and mix in the pureed vegetables and ¾ a cup of ground sunflower seeds. Shape into individual patties. Place into a 350 degree F. oven for 30 minutes, or pan sauté the patties.

HERBED WHITE QUINOA

Use one part grain to two parts vegetable stock or water. Add 1 teaspoon of oregano, 1 teaspoon of thyme, 2 fresh sage leaves and herb or sea salt to taste to the cooking water. Bring to a boil and then simmer for 20 minutes. When the grain is fully cooked, turn off the heat and add 1 chopped sweet red pepper, 1 chopped red onion and 2-3 tablespoons of adzuki beans. Let stand for 5-10 minutes.

GINGERED WILD RICE

Add one part wild rice to two parts vegetable stock and herb or sea salt to taste. Simmer for 30 minutes or until done. Turn off heat and add freshly grated gingerroot and 4-5 artichoke hearts. Cover and let stand for 5 minutes. Garnish with toasted sunflower seeds.

SHANNON'S PASTA WITH SALSA VERDE

Toss together sauteed mushrooms and kale, mix with Tinkyada brown rice pasta and green french lentils, salsa verde.

3 cups loosely packed green herbs (I used flat leaf parsley, cilantro, spinach and basil- other options are sorrel, arugula or watercress)

- 2 cloves garlic
- 2 tablespoon lemon juice
- Pinch of sea salt
- 2 tablespoon capers in brine
- 1/3 cup extra virgin olive oil

Add garlic and salt to food processor(or blender) while it's running. Add herbs and pulse until coarse. With food processor running, add capers, lemon juice and then the olive oil in a slow steady stream. Taste for seasoning, add water, caper brine or more olive oil for a thinner consistency. This sauce is also really great on chicken and beef.

BUTTERNUT SQUASH WITH COCOA

- 1 butternut squash
- 2 tablespoon coconut oil
- 2 tablespoon cacao powder

Prepare the squash by halving it then peeling it. Cut into approximately 1 inch cubes, set in a bowl. In a pan, melt the coconut oil- don't heat it too high, just enough to liquify the oil. Pour melted oil over the squash cubes, tossing them to make sure all are coated. Sprinkle 1 tablespoon of the cocoa over the top of the cubes and toss, sprinkle the rest and toss again until all are evenly coated. Spread cubes onto a parchment lined cooking sheet, cook in a 350 degree F. preheated oven for 30 to 45 minutes.

Snacks

- Nuts & Seeds
- Avocado
- Hummus /Tahini
- Crunchy Veggies (carrots, radish, celery)
- Brown Rice/Lentils/Legumes/ Fruit
- Cucumber with sea salt
- Herbal tea
- Mixed fruit
- Coconut milk smoothie with plum, nectarine, peach, apple
- Nori Chips
- Kale Chips
- Coconut water kefir
- Coconut yogurt
- Avocado with sauerkraut
- Grated, Carrot, Daikon with Nori
- Bone Broth
- Veggie Broth

Drinks

GREEN SMOOTHIE

(Basic) - Everyday - Hydrating, Minerals, Anti-Inflammatory

- 1/2 a bunch dino kale; cut out stalks if not straining
- 1/2 inch ginger
- 5-8 cups water

Optional additions to your green smoothie: apple & kyo-green powder. Pear and mint. Blend up and have with fibers or strain through thin mesh colander.

TEAS

GINGER TEA

Fresh ginger (slice up with skin on) or bagged.

PEPPERMINT / MINT

Fresh mint or bagged.

TURMERIC & GINGER ROOT TEA

- 4-6 cup filtered water
- 2 tablespoon freshly grated ginger root
- 1-2 tablespoon freshly grated turmeric root (or sub 1 teaspoon powder if not available)
- 1 tablespoon fresh lemon juice
- A bit of honey to taste

Bring ginger, turmeric and cayenne almost to boiling in the water. Turn off heat and let sit for 5-10 min. Add lemon juice. Strain into a cup and add honey to taste. You can reuse the mixture more than once adding more water and heating.

DETOX BATH:

- 2 cups of epsom salts plus,
- 2 cups of baking soda
- 0 drops of lavender

DETOX BROTH

- 3 quarts of water
- 1 large chopped onion
- 2 sliced carrots
- 1 cup of daikon or white radish root
- 1 cup of winter squash cut into large cubes
- 1 cup of root veggies (turnips/parsnips and rutabagas for sweetness)
- 2 cups of chopped greens: kale, parsley, beet greens, collard greens, chard, dandelion, cilantro or other greens
- 3 celery stalks
- ½ cup of seaweed: nori, dulse, wakame, kelp or kombu
- ½ cup of cabbage
- 4 ½ inch slices of ginger
- 2 cloves of whole garlic (not chopped or crushed)
- Sea salt to taste

Add all the ingredients at once and place on low boil for 60 minutes. Cool & strain veggies out-discard them. Makes approximately 8 cups. Store in fridge. Simply heat and drink 3-4 cups/day.

Stores

TIP: Shop the outer ring of the super market. Avoid aisles (full of packaged & processed foods)

LOCAL VEGGIES

Health Food Stores

Whole Foods

Farmer's Market

Community Supported Agriculture boxes (CSA)

WHOLE FOODS, FOOD COURT: GLOBAL CUISINE SECTION

- Chicken Chile Verde
- Herb Roast Turkey Breast
- Grilled Veggies
- Steamed veggies
- Black Quinoa Hummus
- Broccoli
- Steamed Brown Rice
- Red Onion
- Cilantro
- Guacamole

CHEF'S CHOICE SECTION

- Carrot & Beet Salad

SALAD BAR

Everything but edamame, corn, cherry tomatoes, salad dressing, eggs, peppers, tofu, tuna, macaroni, orzo salad, chile lime basil tofu, cucumber salad, marinated roasted tomatoes, cheese.

SOUPS

- Chicken veggie
- Spicy vegan pumpkin soup
- Split Pea

Tip: What to order when you're out in a restaurant

- Protein - chicken, fish, lamb, lentils, legumes
- Salad
- Vegetables
- Brown rice/quinoa
- Noodles – rice based

CUISINE TYPES

THAI

Focus on coconut soups, curries

VIETNAMESE

Focus on noodle soups, spring roll

JAPANESE

Focus on sushi, bring your coconut aminos, avoid the tempura

INDIAN

Focus on daal, curries

ANNE'S GLUTEN-FREE FAVORITES:

BREADS & CRACKERS

- Food for Life Rice Breads
- Sesamark Crackers

HOT CEREALS

- Ancient Harvest Quinoa Flakes with almond/hazelnut milk
- Lundberg Brown Rice Cereal with almond/ hazelnut milk

COLD CEREALS

- Fiona's Quinoa Crunch
- Make your own Muesli-with fresh fruit, and 1 scoop of ground flax with sesame/sunflower/pumpkin seed and/or almonds

PASTAS

- Thai rice stick noodles/rice vermicelli noodles
- Brown rice pasta Tinkyada brand

About the Author

Anne Angelone, Licensed Acupuncturist

Bachelor of Science, Cornell University Master of Science, American College of Traditional Chinese Medicine

Member of Primal Docs The Paleo Physician's Network

And Dr. Kharrazian's Thyroid Docs

✦ Background ✦

My own experience with Ankylosing Spondylitis (AS) led me to study the underlying mechanisms of disease expression. Since Ankylosing Spondylitis is correlated with the gene type called HLA B-27, I learned how to identify and remove specific triggers and then how to heal my leaky gut. I also learned how it's possible to turn off inflammatory gene expression with nutrition, supplements, Qi (oxygen), acupuncture, exercise, diet, and meditation. I'm grateful to be able to share what I have learned through experience and years of research, training and investigation.

My background in Functional Medicine has included advanced training with Dr. Datis Kharrazian in Functional Blood Chemistry Analysis, Mastering the Thyroid, Neurotransmitters and the Brain, Functional Endocrinology, Autoimmunity and Gluten Sensitivity

My hope is to share this information with those who would like to treat the underlying causes of "chronic symptoms" and experience greater health sooner than later.

For more info contact: www.anneangelone.com

OTHER TITLES BY ANNE ANGELONE

The Autoimmune Paleo Plan

The Autoimmune Diet

The Paleo Autoimmune Protocol

For more info about my preactice, head over to my website to download my free e-book:

Chinese Medicine In The Modern World

Cheers to your great health,

Anne Angelone, Licensed Acupuncturist

San Francisco, CA

website

www.ingramcontent.com/pod-product-compliance
Lightning Source LLC
Chambersburg PA
CBHW070404290526
45790CB00004B/1630